GOD'S WILL

(A TRUE-LIFE STORY)

NON-FICTION

UCHECHUKWU & OBINNA KALU-ORJI

COPYRIGHT PAGE

All rights reserved. No part of this book may be republished in any form or by any means, including photocopying, scanning or otherwise without prior written permission to the copyright holder.

Copyright © 2022 Obinna Kaluorji

TABLE OF CONTENTS

DEDICATION	5
ABOUT THE BOOK	7
INTRODUCTION	9
CHAPTER ONE – THE GENESIS	11
CHAPTER TWO – THE DISCOVERY	15
CHAPTER THREE – THE CONFIRMATION	21
CHAPTER FOUR – THE CAMP	25
CHAPTER FIVE – THE ENCOUNTER	27
CHAPTER SIX – THE DIALYSIS	36
CHAPTER SEVEN – THE COMPLICATIONS	43
CHAPTER EIGHT – THE APPROVED FUND	53
CHAPTER NINE – THE DONOR	56

CHAPTER TEN – THE TRIP TO INDIA　　　　　　59

CHAPTER ELEVEN – THE KIDNEY TRANSPLANT　　67

CHAPTER TWELVE – THE TRANSPLANT PATIENT　　74

CHAPTER THIRTEEN – THE INDIAN COW ATTACK　　77

CHAPTER FOURTEEN – THE RETURN TO NIGERIAN　　79

CHAPTER FIFTEEN – THE THANKSGIVING AND TESTIMONIES
　　　　　　　　　　　　　　　　　　　　　　　　99

CHAPTER SIXTEEN – THE GLORIOUS END　　105

APPRECIATION　　　　　　　　　　　　　　　114

DEDICATION

I would like to dedicate this book to the following persons for the role they played to the existence of this book;

In loving memory of Uchechukwu Kalu-Orji (my brother): Uchechukwu hand wrote this piece himself. Uchechukwu is the reason for this book. He was the person that went through everything that you will see and read in this book. He was documenting all his experience as he was going through all of them. He is the person that hand wrote this book from introduction to appreciation. He titled and mentioned all the names in this book himself. Without him, this book can never be complete and would never have existed.

My mum: My mum single handedly trained us (5 boys) and saw us through school after our dad left us at an early age. The pressure of the demise of my brother (Uchechukwu) was more on her.

Without my mum in the picture, this book would probably be incomplete.

My brothers: My brothers played an important role to the existence of this book. I want to thank my brothers for the love and support they showered on my brother (Uchechukwu) especially bro. Akachi who voluntarily accepted to donate his kidney to him.

That was a brave move and I respect him for that.

My Aunties and my uncles: My aunties and uncles contributed to the success of this book at one point or the other. They were there to help and support my brother and they helped to fast track my brothers travel to India for a kidney transplant.

The Executive governor: The executive governor of our state as at 2005 played an important role to the existence of this book. Without him, this book would probably not have up to the last chapter.

My Friends: My friends played an important role in the life of my brother Uchechukwu. They were there to support and encourage him and they never ceased in their prayers.

My church: My church never ceased in their prayers. They gave my brother the reason to hold and never to give up on life.

ABOUT THE BOOK

The book "God's will" is a non-fiction story of my brother who suffered from kidney disease that later escalated to a kidney failure.

All the name of the persons or places mentioned in this book are real names and real places that exist in the Eastern part of Nigeria.

As requested by my brother, while reading this book, allow the Holy spirit to minister to you. Don't be in a hurry while reading the book. Relax and concentrate while on the book. The book was hand written by my brother Uchechukwu Kalu-Orji while I fine-tuned, modified, typed and published the book but still maintaining the name of persons and places used by my brother Uchechukwu (the writer).

The name of the book "**God's will**" is the name that was intended by my brother Uchechukwu (the writer) as seen in the book's introduction page. If you are opportune to get and read this book, I encourage you to also get for your brothers and sisters because the story is a touchy and real-life story that will encourage you, educate you, correct you, sharpen you, prepare you for the future and ultimately prepare you for the kingdom of God.

My brother that hand wrote the book "**God's will**" is now late but since he intended to publish this book at one point or the other before his demise, I had to make his wish come to reality by publishing it. Having gone through the handwritten version of the book, I found the need to publish the book because I am sure it will be a great piece of information to someone.

I encourage you to take this story as a story told you from heaven and not to joke with the contents. The writer wrote it himself when it was happening to him. On my part, I corrected any English I feel is not correct, typed, published and made the book available on the platform where you could access it.

You are free to share and print this book as many times as you want for personal use but you are not permitted to reproduce this book in any form or use the book for any commercial purpose. Unauthorized use of this book or its content shall be considered as illegal and copyright infringement.

INTRODUCTION

My name is Uchechukwu Kaluorji. I am 17 years old and presently in S.S. 3. I am the last child of my parents. My Dad is late and my Mum single handedly trained us up till this moment. I am from Eastern part of Nigeria. The year I started this writeup is 2004.

This book "GOD'S WILL" was written by Ucheckukwu Kaluorji, to reveal the fact that there is nothing that God cannot do and that in every situation, give thanks to the Almighty God.

This is a story of how I almost died but the Almighty God sustained me all through and today I am alive and healthy. Amen

I want to appreciate the name of the Almighty God who afforded me the opportunity to write this book by giving me life. Also, I worship and praise him for giving me the wisdom with which I used in writing this book and for helping me to remember everything that happened to me about 3 and half years ago. May his name be blessed in Jesus name. Amen.

I want to use this opportunity to thank God for making me to belong to Scripture Union. It is a fellowship where agape love reigns and the peace of God is abundant. They were there for me by the grace of God. I want to thank God for these people – Ugochi, Nnenna and the excos of 2005/2006 session. May God bless them all. I want to also thank my twin brother Obinna, Ogonna, Friday, Oluchi, Nkechi, Ogbuzuru and my sisters Ifeoma, Nkiru and Alice. May God bless you all, Amen.

CHAPTER ONE – The Genesis

This is a story of how I suffered from a kidney infection which later grew into a kidney failure almost to the point of death but God sustained my life till today. When you read this story, allow the Holy Spirit to minister to you.

It all started in the year 2002 When I was in J.S.S 3A. In my second term, early February, when we were preparing for our Junior exam, I found out that I was feeling weak inside but I thought it was normal. Sometimes, I will come back from school and after keeping my bag and removing my uniform, I will go and sleep for 4-5 hours without waking up and this continued for some time. My Mum noticed and asked if I was sick and I will just say "Nothing" but the truth was that I never knew what was wrong with me.

Little did we know that it was an early stage of kidney infection. It grew to a point that I started spitting (vomiting saliva) in every 1 or 2 minutes and nobody knew what was wrong. I started losing appetite and I couldn't eat well and nobody knew that the kidney was getting bad. It was not diagnosed on time and the organ was getting bad.

One day, that was on Sunday, my cousin that was living with us and that took care of us when we were young by name Ukachi, noticed that my face was changing to another complexion (White) and that my face was a little bit swollen. She went and told my Mum and my Mum was confused and surprised. That Sunday evening, my Mum had to take me to a doctor. The doctor was from my village by name Dr Okoro. We went to his house and he examined me that day and also confirmed that I was very weak and he advised my Mum to be giving me beverages because I was losing fluid through the vomiting of saliva and we agreed. He also told us to come to the hospital where he was works the next day being a Monday.

On Monday morning. I didn't go to school on time even though we had a class exam. That day, we went to the Federal Medical Center, went to the doctor's office and saw him but he old us that the doctor seeing people of my age was not on seat (I was around 14-15 years by then) and that we should come again. After we must have paid for our card and folder file, he took us to the laboratory for a urine and blood test. After the test, they told us (I and my Mum) to come back in the next 2-3 days and they more they delayed, the more the kidney grew worse.

We came back 3 days later and Dr Okoro told us again that my doctor as not on seat that day but he saw the result of the test and told my Mum that I had sugar, blood, albumin and so many other things in my urine and these are the nutrients that should be filtered by my kidney but it was not filtered and it was coming out through my Urine which was an indication that my kidneys were bad. The doctor did not make us to understand it well but told us to come the next day and see my doctor.

The next day being around Friday, we went to the hospital again and still did not see the doctor.

Dear reader, we went to the hospital for almost two weeks and the doctor was not around. Even the drugs Dr Okoro prescribed for me to reduce the vomiting, instead of taking them, I was throwing them away and will pretend as if I have taken them. I never knew that I was doing myself more harm than good. In these two weeks, my kidneys were getting worse by the day. One day, we went to the hospital and met a doctor (woman). After looking at the result of my test, she told us that the hospital had no equipment like ultrasound machine to continue with the medication and that we should go to the teaching hospital. We went home disappointed.

On Sunday afternoon, my Mum phoned my uncle by name Uche who lived at Enugu and he told us to come to his location before it got worse. That same day in the evening, we were already in his house from where we intend to go the hospital.

CHAPTER TWO – The Discovery

On that same day (Sunday), we went to a hospital and that evening my Mum started everything afresh. We started by purchasing our card which was #750 by then and since that day was not a working day, we had to pay another #1000 for emergency.

We wanted to see an Indian doctor by name doctor Picado but the nurse on duty that night by name nurse Ujunwa told my uncle that the doctor he wanted to see was not on seat that night and that it was only one Dr Chigbo that was on seat. My uncle and his wife alongside my Mum agreed to see the doctor for that night on knowing the fact that the nurse promised us that we will see the Indian doctor the next day. We went in and told him our problems which he wrote down in a folder as report and said I should be placed on admission. My Mum made a deposit of #15000 for a private room where I was taken to. Later that night, my uncle`s wife prepared a meal which was served to me, and after eating I slept off. My Mum couldn't sleep throughout the night (what a caring mother)

The next day (Monday), the Indian doctor came to my room and examined me. He took my blood sample and my urine for test, and gave me drugs. Series of tests and ultrasound were carried out for complete three days, and on Thursday I was discharged

On that same day, the doctor told my Mum that I had a kidney infection called "glomerulus nephritis". My Mum didn't understand of course it was in medical term. He explained further saying it is the inflammation of the nephrons of the kidney caused by bacteria. This nephron is like a filter in the kidney which does not allow some nutrients to pass through urine. It filters the urine, separating the nutrients from the urine but unfortunately mine has been affected. This simply means that the important nutrients like protein, blood, sugar, salt and every other thing cannot be reabsorbed by the kidney and therefore they keep passing out through urine, which made me weaker day by day.

By the time we were discharged from the hospital, the swelling stopped, and we were given some drugs and was told to be coming for checkup, at least every month. So, we went back home. My twin Obinna who was very worried was so happy. We ate together, took my drugs and slept off.

After about 1-2 weeks, I found out my whole body began to swell up which include my face, shoulders, chest and legs. It was called **oedema** which is a sign showing that someone has kidney problem. We went to the hospital again for checkup at Enugu, where some tests were conducted, and the doctor said my cholesterol level was high. I was also given some drugs and was told to come again. Each checkup, we also spend nothing less than #2000, but GOD was so faithful to my family and I.

During that period, my classmate and strangers will be making mockery of me, some of my friends started running away from me thinking I had a communicable disease. Even some teachers were terrified because I grew so fat. Little did they know it wasn't ordinary fatness but swelling due to the kidney infection, but when they got to know, they had pity on me. I can never forget some teachers like Mrs. Nwoye, Mrs. Ewa, and some other teachers. Who advised me and told me to be prayerful and also remind God of his promises in my life, especially Mrs. Nwoye. She always pampered me as if I'm her child. In school, she wouldn't allow me do any hard work because she knew it will definitely affect me. I pray that may God bless these two teachers for me in Jesus name, Amen.

Because of the swellings, I was still going for checkup at Enugu to see the Indian doctor and he was still giving me drugs. Each time he gave me drugs, the swellings will tend to reduce but if the drugs finish, it will return and personally I was confused.

One day being a Monday in the year 2003, I went for checkup with my Mum and we went to see this experienced doctor from India but to my surprise, the doctor said something "this disease cannot be cured here but can be managed; you have to look for a nephrologist who would take care of him". When he said this, I behaved as if I did not hear it and after everything, I asked my Mum what he said but she simply said "nothing" maybe because she never wanted it to bother me. That day, we went home disappointed.

One day, the wife of our landlord by name Mrs. Okafor told us that there was a nephrologist at Enugu, she gave us the address of the clinic but the main address was not correct and my Mum never knew the place. My Mum (a secondary school principal) contacted one of her teachers and told her about our predicament and showed her the address that our landlords wife gave us. Due to the fact that she was living at Enugu, she knew her way around and could be of help to us. She decided to help us and that afternoon, we set off to Enugu to look for the clinic.

When we got to Enugu, we went to so many clinics (about 5 of them) and search of that particular clinic. Our vehicle spoilt on the way but by the grace of God, it was repaired and we started looking for the clinic again. As God may have it, the 5th clinic we went to gave us the correct address of the clinic we were looking for. We went to the new address and got to the clinic in the evening around 4pm.

We sat down and waited for the doctor because it was an evening clinic. In the course of the waiting, the teacher said that she wanted to go and my Mum wanted to appreciate her by giving her some money which she refused and we thanked her for her

help and she departed. Finally, the doctor arrived but before we could see him, we had to start all over again by buying card and other things but this one was more expensive. After the purchase, we sat down and waited for our turn.

CHAPTER THREE – The Confirmation

Before it got to our turn to see the doctor, it was already 6pm in the evening. When we entered the doctor's office, we greeted the doctor and the doctor took report. The doctor ran some tests that evening (blood and urine tests) and he also gave me a gallon for me to put my 24 hours urination. The cost of the tests was about #15,0000 and he also gave us drugs of about #9,000. When I saw the cost, I had pity on my Mum and I started blaming myself for being sick but it was not my fault and I still believed that God wanted to do something with me.

That evening, we went back to my uncle's house as it was already late and since we need to get the report of the tests and also complete my 24 hours urination exercise, we could not go back to our base but stayed back at Enugu. In the evening (the following day), we went back to the clinic and saw the doctor. After examining the result of the tests, the doctor said that I had **glomerulus nephritis** which was a confirmation in accordance to what the first doctor said. He gave us a paper and told us to go for ultrasound at Hansa clinic the next day.

The next day, we went to hansa clinic with my uncle Uche; we paid for the ultrasound (about #1500). My Mum wanted to go to school that day, so she went out before the ultrasound and told my uncle to bring me back.

I finished the ultrasound and got the report but I waited for my uncle for about 3-4 hours. Since my uncle did not show up after 3-4 hours, I thought he forgot so I had to start going back to our house as my Mum gave me some money before she left. By the grace of God, I boarded a bus and came back to our house safely.

The next day, in the evening we had to go back again to the clinic to show the report of the ultrasound to the Doctor. He examined it and told us the level of the damage and also sent us for a blood test that night (around 8pm). After the test, we bought drugs prescribed by the doctor before going back to my uncles' house that night.

The next day, we went back to the clinic in the evening as usual. After seeing the doctor, my Mum told him our predicament (driving at night and the cost of the drugs).

My Mum asked him if we could him at the teaching hospital because that was where he works as a consultant and he agreed. My Mum was a little bit relieved and we went back home. The next day we went to Teaching Hospital Enugu as we discussed with the doctor and as usual, we purchased card and waited for our turn. When it came to our turn, we went in to see the doctor but to our surprise, he behaved as if he has never seen us up to a point that my Mum had to ask him if he really knew us and he simply said "yes". We were even thinking that maybe he is angry that we did not come to his private clinic.

He prescribed some drugs and gave us to buy in the hospital but we thought that it would e costly in the hospital, so we bought it at our location where we think it should be less expensive. Because of the way the hospital treated us, we had to switch to our former Hospital.

I started checkups again at the Hospital and they were managing the kidney infection. God was protecting and guiding me as I went for checkups alone. I went TO and FRO the hospital almost every two weeks and God was protecting me. For went for checkups for many months still the swellings were there. I was still going for checkups believing God that one day he would touch me.

One thing I want to make you to understand dear reader, is that these things happening were the will of God and we must learn how to allow the will of God to be done in our lives and we will never regret it in Jesus' name, Amen. Sometimes I will ask my brother why I should be the last to be born and still be the first to die in my family, and I know that it was a negative confession, God forgive me.

Sometimes I will go behind the curtain and start crying and my cousin by name Nnenna will console and pray for me. People like my twin brother Obinna, Ogonna, Otuu, Nkechi, Ifeoma were there for me.

CHAPTER FOUR – The Camp

I was still going for checkups at Enugu until August that year. We had to go for our Scripture Union Student camp. The camp was beautiful with the theme of the year being "The Scripture". We spent 4 days learning about the bible- Its power, its use and how to use it while praying.

On the last day, in the evening was our variety night that everyone was supposed to dance, give testimonies and special numbers. With my heart full of joy, I was dancing and praising God. Our fellow-up secretary for that year by name bro Ogonna touched me and pointed at some girls. I looked at the girls and to my surprise, these girls were looking and laughing at me and immediately my countenance changed automatically. This made me not to dance throughout that night for I said to myself "If my classmates who were unbelievers laughed at me and now those that are supposed to be my sisters are also laughing at me, then I am finished"

The next day we went back home and few days later, the swelling began to reduce to a point that people thought that I was alright. I also concluded that I was alright and because of that, I reduced the rate of going for checkup forgetting that faith without work is dead. I was moving around freely with my friends who also thought that I was now alright. I went as far as giving testimony in one of our night vigils, telling them that I was alright and they were all happy and praised the Lord with me. In my family everyone was happy that the swelling reduced forgetting that it was internal (kidney). Some weeks later I found out that sometimes, my heart or chest will be as if it is trying to compress and I will be very weak. Sometimes, I will be sweating but I will pretend as if I was okay. I said to myself that the sign was just a manipulation from the pit of hell.

In the year 2004 by September, I had a companion and friend who helped both in my spiritual life and physical life and by the grace of God, I will never forget her. Anytime it started happening to me, she would notice and will be asking me if I was okay. I would tell her what was wrong with me and she would advice and encourage me telling me that everything would be alright and that God would see me through. After our exams, I took pictures with some of my classmates and we vacated for the first term and that was the second week of December. We said bye to ourselves and parted for Christmas.

CHAPTER FIVE – The Encounter

On 23rd of December, we travelled to the village and I never knew what that year December held for me. I was moving around freely until around 27th December 2002. I started being very weak. All the time I would be sleeping, lost appetite and my mouth became sour almost all the time. My uncle by name uncle Chibuike who based at Abia then, told me to be eating not as food but as drug. According to him, the cause of my weakness was lack of food.

It continued that way until 1st January 2005. Early in the morning around 6am, I found out that my mouth was very heavy and I thought it was saliva. I went outside to vomit what was in my mouth but to my greatest surprise, it was blood. I was afraid to tell my Mum because I knew how she would react to it rather I called my elder brother who is studying medicine and surgery at the state university. When he saw it, he was a little bit scared and he went in and called my Mum and on seeing it, she started crying bitterly telling God to deliver me.

She opened the year with crying but I still believed that she would close the year with joy. All the attempt to console her failed. My brother tried to explain to her that my tongue was broken because my blood count was low and Mum asked why it was low. The explanation was that a part of the kidney which helps the bone marrow to produce blood was affected due to the fact that I had kidney problem.

My Mum was supposed to go for a meeting which she decided not to go again, but my uncle persuaded her to go, while they took care of me. My brother and uncle took me to maternal uncle Dr. Ogbonna. He was working in a teaching hospital. After meeting with him, he discovered I was looking so pale, and said the exact thing my brother said about the blood count being low because of the kidney problem. He advised I should be taking glucose, so it could give me energy for some time.

On the 10th of January 2005 was school resumption, so we came back on the 5th to get prepared. Everything was going so well until 9th of January being Sunday. I was in the church when I started having some strange feelings.

I started feeling cold and shivering at the same time, to the extent I couldn't answer any question during Sunday school, but I had to manage to stay throughout the service. My Mum couldn't drive us home because of the meeting she had, so she gave my brother and I some money to take tricycle. When we got home, we ate and rested. When Mum got home, she ordered me to wash plates, and when doing so I noticed I was becoming weak, though my Mum noticed but she wasn't sure of my behavior.

After washing the plates, I quickly went in to lay down, my Mum noticed my movement and followed me in asking if I'm ok, but I couldn't respond. She quickly called my elder brother. Immediately, I was rushed to our assistant pastor's house that evening for prayers, but unfortunately, he was not in. Rev. Jospeh saw me and rendered a short prayer. He assured my Mum that I would be ok. So, my Mum also took me to another Reverend by name Victor, on getting there, we found out that he wasn't in, so we met with his daughter Nkiru who brought out mat for me to lay on.

While waiting, Mum bought lucozade boost to know if it could give me some energy, which I took. Rev Aghachi came back and saw me laying down, and out of curiosity he asked what was wrong, which Mum narrated everything to him.

He prayed stupendously and commanded me to stand with my feet that I'm healed, and lo and behold I stood praise God!

We went home that day; I was still taking the Lucozade boost and I was alright. About an hour later, our paster rev. okey and an elder of the church – elder Charles visited me. The pastor who prayed for me earlier in the day confirmed that I was alright because I could now talk. In the evening, I ate and slept on the bed with my twin brother (Obinna). In the night around 1 am, the thing started again but this time it was serious. If I stretch my legs, it would be shaking repeatedly and my brother wanted to cry. If I look at my brother, I couldn't focus on him though I try to. I was crying, my twin brother (Obinna) was cleaning my tears and begged me to sleep. He was pampering me like a child, singing for me so that I could sleep (what a loving brother).

It was happening like that till around 3 am in the morning, my elder brother by name Chima came out to urinate and heard me cry. He came inside the room and saw how serious it was, he alerted everybody in the family. My Mum on seeing me became more confused but Akachi told her to calm down. My brothers asked me what was wrong with me, I could not talk rather I was laughing. Bro Chima turned to my twin brother and started blaming him for not alerting everybody on time but rather stayed and was doing it alone but in defense, my brother (Obinna) said that he never wanted to disturb anyone that night.

Around 5am that morning, my elder brother Chima backed me into our landlord's car and we went to a doctor's house (Mrs. Mercy). We woke the doctor up and she gave me an injection and some drugs and told us to come to the hospital the next day for some tests.

When we got home that Monday morning being 10th January, my Mum wanted to give me a cup of tea to drink but unfortunately, I had already lost my appetite but I tried

to drink the tea with straw after much persuasions from my Mum and my landlord's wife. Our school was supposed to re-open that day but I didn't go but rather we went to mercy hospital as discussed earlier. When we got to the hospital, we saw the doctor and after checking my blood pressure, she asked my Mum if I was anemic and my Mum said No (because my blood pressure was high).

She ran some tests in me and told my Mum that I would be on a bed so that I could take a drip and that we had to wait for the report of the tests. I was on drip and my Mum went to school to tell them what made her not to come to school on the first day of reopening. In her absence, something terrible happened. After 30 minutes, I started reacting to the drip they gave me. I was shouting and crying and after sometime I would be unconscious, my face wanted to go to the back and my bones stiffened. Everybody was confused including the doctor.

They called the reaction "RIGOUR", the doctor had to change the drip before I was alright. I wanted to see my twin brother and my Mum brought him for me and he saw me, he was extremely happy that I was alright.

The next day being Tuesday 11th January, I was still on admission in the hospital. The result of the tests came out and after examining them, the doctor told us that I had "Cerebral Malaria" which meant that the malaria entered my brain. She gave us some drug and discharged me but she said I should come every day for checkup. We got home and relaxed but later in the day, a family friend and a doctor – Dr. Benjamin came around. He said that if cerebral malaria is not detected on time, you could make someone to go mad or die and I thanked God that my own was noticed on time. In addition, my elder brother Dr Emeka said that was why I was just laughing I.E I lost my memory. We went for checkup on Wednesday and Thursday, the doctor told us to go to Enugu the next day to know the level of the kidney damage. She gave us a letter stating how far she went and the things wrong with me.

On Friday 14th January 2005, we set out to Enugu. When it got to our turn after about 3 hours of waiting, we went in to see the doctor but this time, it was Dr. Eze. We gave him the letter and after reading it, he examined me by opening my eyes. He said I was pale and very weak and that I should be placed on admission because I was too weak to be coming to the hospital from the house. My Mum agreed and paid a deposit of #15,000 for a private room and unfortunately, according to the nurses, there was no private room available. After waiting for about 2 hours to see if any private room would be available but to no avail. They decided to put in a general room, the number of the room was 10b. When I got to the room, I was disgusted by the kind of people I saw there. They were like that are expecting death anytime but I had no choice but to stay in the room.

To my surprise, they were not giving adequate care rather they were fixing drip one after the other. I couldn't eat and if I tried to eat, I would vomit even the one I did not eat. It came to a point that I vomited and my vomit was green in color.

In addition to this, I was going to toilet in every 5 – 10 minutes and my stool would be blackish green in color because there was no food in my stomach. I was getting thinner and weaker by the day. They were giving me drugs and I vomited most of them. I could not eat; I could not take some of my drugs and I was vomiting.

CHAPTER SIX – The Dialysis

On Saturday 15 January 2005, a tragic thing happened in the evening. I was not breathing very well again because blood blocked my nose, my eyes wanted to turn white and my tongue that was supposed to be wet became dry and black in color. The fact is that I almost died that night around 9pm. Seeing everything that was happening, my Mum was very confused and scared. She was praying seriously, shouting the blood of Jesus. That day was the first day I went for dialysis (**Dialysis** is the removal of wastes from the blood. Dialysis does the work of kidney to the body if the kidney is damaged). My uncle earlier told my Mum that I would go for dialysis on Monday but now the situation was out of hand and if nothing was done about it, I might die. My Mum wanted to call my uncle but there was no service and she became more confused but praise the lord a miracle happened – (That dialysis center does not open after they have closed by 7.30pm but this was around 10pm in the night. My uncle tried to tell them how serious the situation was but they insisted we come on Monday.

My uncle connected to a high person by name prof. Ama. Prof. Ama connected those people that were to do it, told them to do it that night. Meanwhile, my uncle was supposed to go for a conference but God kept him back, if not, nobody knew what could have happened because my Mum knew nothing about the dialysis and she was confused). My uncle called us and told us to prepare that the dialysis was that night and more on Monday. On hearing this, my Mum was a little bit relieved but she was still praying seriously for me. My uncle later arrived with is jeep and I was carried with a stretcher into the car because I couldn't walk. When we got to the hospital, the nurses tried to stop us but I was not possible for them. We went for the dialysis and they told us that we had to pay #30,000 for registration, #25,000 for dialysis and #11,000 for two piles of blood making it a total of #61,000 just for that night but my Mum still in confusion did not listen to them. As God may have it, my uncle rev Uche paid the money and I was dialyzed and given blood.

By 2am, I was still on dialysis machine and after the dialysis at about 2.35am on Sunday morning, we went back to the hospital, but remember that in the course of the dialysis, the toilet tissue that my mum finished while she was using it to clean the blood that was coming out of my nose and mouth.

I also vomited saliva and digested food in my stomach throughout the dialysis and also reacted to the blood transfusion. I was shouting and crying, I even wanted to stand up with the tube full of my blood which was life threatening, 4 men tried to hold me but they could not until my uncle rev Uche had to ask me why I was behaving like someone that is possessed. He also reminded me that peoples life depends on it. After sometime, still on the machine, my tongue started coming out automatically and we told the doctor dialyzing me by name doctor Obinna and his nurse – Nurse Patricia but he started laughing and called it a reaction. He said it was normal and that it would be okay.

When we finally finished, I was carried to the car and on our way back, my tongue started coming out again. My Mum was walked up and she called my uncle to look at me but my uncle being full of faith told her that I was alright. When we got to the hospital, they had already closed everywhere but as God may have it, a nurse came out and brought a wheel chair and they took me to my room and I laid down. I could not sleep because my head was turning to the back automatically. Each time it happens, I would call my Mum who was fast asleep to come and turn it to normal because it was paining me but I could not turn it myself.

My Mum would wake up and help me turn my head to normal for me. I started having pity for my Mum because for some time, she was not going to work and she was also getting thinner because of the worry and pressure put on her and I blame myself for being sick. I know one thing that I would pay her back in the future since she allowed God to use to give me back my life "GOD BLESS HER".

On that same morning around 4am, I wanted to go to toilet with my drip but I never wanted to disturb my Mum, I went on my own but after going to the toilet, I stood up and automatically, I bent to the back and it was paining me but I could not help it. I did not know how to call my Mum, I weas there for almost 2-3 minutes and I started crying before a boy also in the same room came and stretched me and that was when my Mum came and asked me why I went alone. I told her that I never wanted to disturb her and she told me to be disturbing her and that it was why she was there (God must bless my Mum).

In the morning around 7am that Sunday, the automatic turning of the head also continued and each time, I would still call my Mum but she was uncomfortable with it. Around 9am that morning, the doctor came for ward round and we told him but to my surprise, he did not take any critical strategy to stop it but he went his way. That morning, they gave me food that was tasteless and I could not eat but begged my Mum to eat it for me but unfortunately, her own stomach was tied up because I have not eaten.

In fact, the hospital was not taking care of me adequately, and we didn't know why. It was later my uncle discovered that the room we were staying was the place they keep people that were expected to die anytime, and in other words, they were waiting for me to give up to ghost. Mercy said no, because it wasn't the will of God for me.

On that Sunday afternoon, my brothers visited me. Bro Emeka, bro Chima, bro Nnachi, my cousin and his mum also came around also. I requested to see my twin brother Obinna, and was told he didn't come but would come later. I was sad because I haven't seen him for some time.

On Monday being 17th of January, I was discharged and we went to dialysis again, we paid #20,000 and I was dialyzed. I was crying because I remembered what happened to me on the first day, but this one was better than the last one, though very painful. While on the machine, I couldn't see clearly nor hear very well, but I was hearing noises in my ear.

Dialysis is the process of filtering or purifying the blood of waste product which will be filtered by the kidney. I had kidney failure, so kidney infection grew into kidney failure. While filtering, it means that blood would be taken out of one body and enters into the machine, and returned back to the body which you make you feel better (2-3 days)

After the dialysis that Monday afternoon, we went to my uncle's house, and on 18th of January, my elder bro Akachi came and I asked after my twin brother, he told me he would come the following day, and I was a bit relived.

On Tuesday evening around 4pm, I became restless and uncomfortable, I started crying and shouting, and this was caused by high concentration of Uremia in the blood also as a result of kidney failure.

Uremia is a symptom showing that someone has kidney failure. On Wednesday 19th, we went to dialysis again, but before then I refused to go because of the pains, my mum pleaded with me. Who am I to say no to my precious mother, even though I know it wouldn't be an easy one, and also don't want her to be sad, So I had to give in. We went and God helped me, so we headed home to my uncle's place.

CHAPTER SEVEN – The Complications

On Wednesday afternoon, my twin brother came and was extremely happy to see me. We talked and he told me everything that have been happening in school, and I also told him about my experiences. So, we were taken to Mr. Biggs, and we ate and ate.

The next day being Thursday 20th January, we went to my home town, and my friends and classmates came to pray for me. On Monday 24th January, the restlessness came back. I was so restless and uncomfortable, so my twin brother didn't go to school that day because he was taking care of me. I would sit down and lie down 10 times in 2 minutes due to the restlessness. All thanks to my twin bro Obinna because he has been of great help to me. He would prefer to be uncomfortable just for me to be comfortable, and anytime I cry, he would cry with me (what a loving brother. I know that one day I would pay him for what he allowed God to use him to do). On Tuesday, I went for dialysis and after that we went back to the Ijeoma clinic. We told the doctor our experience for the past two weeks and he wrote it down. He sent us for a blood test and told us to go for ultrasound the next day at hansa clinic.

We did it as instructed and came back the next day in the evening. He saw the results both the blood test and the result of the ultrasound, then confirmed that I had kidney failure. He gave us drugs and told us to be coming for checkups.

     Since kidney failure cannot be cured except by Renal Replacement Therapy (R.R.T) which includes dialysis and kidney transplant, there was need to source for fund. We needed money for kidney transplant because dialysis was not the best option. The kidney transplant was costly and there was no money but another miracle happened. The money for my dialysis, no one knows where it was coming from. People were giving us money to help – Scripture Union, Assemblies of God church, SS 3 students of our set and other private individuals etc. In addition to this, a greater miracle happened. My uncle rev Uche came and announced to us that the governor of our state has approved a sum of money for the kidney transplant and also, he approved 250k to help in my dialysis before the travelling. Initially, they wanted to fly me to Germany for the transplant but it was expensive so the agreed to fly me to India which was less expensive.

By now my uncle by name Okey who based at Lagos came down to where we were to help my Mum and to also help in pursuing the formalities of the money already approved. My aunty who based at Lagos by name Ngozi also came to help out in encouraging my Mum and keep her company.

After seeing Dr. Ijeoma, we went home and, in few weeks, I grew from one complication to another which include swelling of the tip of the hand because of lack of protein (Doctor in the hospital told me not to take protein filled foods and it was paining me). I could not hear very well (sometimes I would stay in a closed room and be crying and shouting because of it), I could not see very well (in fact, my eyes were turning that I couldn't watch television), pains all around my neck (that is, I could not turn my neck to any direction), I could not sit down and I could not stand up, I could not lie on my back, buttocks, chest, legs, muscles of the hands and legs. I could not do anything on my own that is, I could not go to toilet, take my bath, walk, some time eat, sleep, stay on my own. Its either my twin brother was there or I will start crying like a baby.

Because of these complications, especially the discomfort and restlessness which disturbed everybody in the house, I went for dialysis in every three days (#20,000 for each time).

For several weeks, we were waiting for the money approved by the government but unfortunately, they delayed due to protocols of the government which meant that we had to be going for dialysis until they release the fund. As God may have it, the 250k approved for my dialysis was released to us.

This period was when I knew I was loved by so many people both in school, church and in the scripture union fellowship including my close friends and classmates. I will not stay a day without them visiting and praying for me, crying unto God on my behalf. I cannot finish calling all their names now but I can't help calling some of them. I can't forget these people – Ugochi and her sister Amarachi, Nnenna, Oluchi, Nkechi, Nkiruka, Alice, my sister Ifeoma and so many others that I can't remember their names and I can never forget my twin brother – Obinna Kaluorji.

These people were there all the time encouraging me, praying for and keeping me company. I want to remember my church – they came almost all Sundays to pray for me both the men and women. I want also remember SS3 students who visited, encouraged and game me some money in addition to what the church gave me.

Also, my uncles – okey and Chibuike, my aunty – Ngozi were all there helping my Mum in all section e.g., encouragements.

The complications later grew to breathlessness i.e. I could not breath well again. We went to Dr Ijeoma and told him about the complications, he said it was caused by the excess fluid in my body which wants to block my chest/lungs and that we should go for dialysis.

He also told us that when it starts, that I should sit upright to enable the fluid flow down to my legs and not my lungs but he did not tell me to reduce water intake since it was caused by excess fluid and ignorantly, I was taking much water. The water that took makes it to return in a short time and everyone was wondering why.

The government people delayed us for a long time and the money given to us was finishing by every 2 days (for dialysis). On one Sunday afternoon, the women of our church came and prayed for me seriously and went home.

To our surprise, in the night the breathlessness came back again but this time, it was serious, if I sit down like the doctor said. I will still be there and lying down was worse.

That night, I was taken to the state teaching hospital and I placed on oxygen for some time but it did not help me and I told them to remove it. As God may have it on the next day, I went for dialysis at Enugu after which I took an injection. The injection costs about #6,000 and we went back home.

On Tuesday, in the evening, we went nephrologist Ijeoma and told him what happened. He looked at my hand eyes and said I was pale and that I needed blood and we agreed. On Wednesday, we went for the dialysis, my mum bought 2 piles of blood, and the first pile was used on me. So, my uncle and mum went to see how much the British airline would cost, while my aunty was with me. After the first pile, the second was used on me, and in the next 5-10 minutes, I started reacting to it. I couldn't breathe very well, my whole body started shaking. I was covered with two blankets, but suddenly I started feeling burning sensation on my chest. My aunty was confused, but being a prayerful woman, she started praying for me. She held every part of my body calling the "blood of Jesus". I nearly died, but saved me again.

Dr. Obinna came and checked my back using stethoscope and shouted saying that air wasn't entering my back. He quickly collected money from my aunty to buy injection, the nurse herself was confused because she was just looking at my aunty who was still praying.

Suddenly, the machine stopped on its own, the nurse tried to revive it but to no avail. She thought it was the electricity, though there was light.

Also, there was another woman who was also dialyzed. She quickly sent her daughter Chidimma to go and put on the generator, and she came with the news that the key to the generator broke inside of it (devil is indeed a liar)

The blood inside the tube started turning black, and the nurse had to disconnect me temporally. The doctor came back with the injections, and gave me one for the cold and also one for the breathlessness, though it continued for sometimes and reduced. Immediately, my mum and uncle came back and started panicking, but my aunty was busy thanking GOD, because she saw what happened. So, when we went home, I couldn't eat because I was still recovering from the psychological trauma. Later I recovered and ate.

On Saturday, we went to dialysis again and waited for the doctor, and when we saw him, we were told the machine wasn't working. Though I was a bit strong, so we had to go back home unattended. So, on Monday, we went back to enugu for the dialysis.

While on the dialysis, the Nepa light was unrestored and the small generator was on which couldn't bring light, and it was in the night but can temporally hold the machine.

They had to bring candle to check something around the machine which was very dangerous and life threatening. So, the doctor said I should be disconnected so that my blood would be able to roll back. The dialysis was supposed to be 3 hours, but was about 1hr 20 minutes, and the hospital promised to compensate when next we come. My mum, uncle and aunty were devastated and promised never to go there again for dialysis, so they decided to take me to Lagos in order to continue my dialysis.

So, on Thursday, we left, on getting to enugu, the breathlessness started so we called Dr. Obinna to see if it could be done in his hospital in enugu, but unfortunately, he wasn't in town. I told my mum that I can manage till we get to Lagos.

On getting to Onitsha, it grew worse and serious that I couldn't breathe at all, to the extent of asking my mum what to do. My mum was afraid and started shouting.

My uncle stopped the car, and everyone came out to pray for me, and after that, they quickly turn back to enugu. So, we went to Dr. Ijeoma clinic that morning to see if they could do anything. The nurse suggested the injection that would be given to me, she said further that the doctor wasn't around, that he went to river state for a conference, which Dr. Obinna also went. So, one of the nurses called another doctor to see if she could give me that injection, and the doctor said NO.

I was so weak that I couldn't walk, my twin brother had to back me, so we walked away disappointed. The breathlessness grew worse, so in the center of confusion, we didn't know what else to do and as God may have it, my aunty suggested we called dr. Obinna again, which we did, so he told us that he would arrange for a doctor, but according to him, the problem was how to convince the nurse because she was in the working place. He told us to try convincing her. So, we thanked him and went to see the nurse again, and she told us to wait for her in the dialysis center, that she would come by 1:30pm.

So, we waited until past 2pm, and she showed up and was arranging things for my dialysis, so when the doctor (Dr. Chukwu) arrived, he asked my mum to buy blood for transfusion, which she did and it was a success this time. I was now very strong and the next day being Friday, we finally travelled to Lagos.

CHAPTER EIGHT – The approved fund

Remember that the governor of our state approved some money for my transplant and also gave us the sum of 250k for my dialysis till we finally travel, we've been using the 250k ever since and it's almost about to finish. The money we were waiting for the kidney transplant has not been signed due to how Dr. Ijeoma delayed in writing a reference letter to be signed by the governor, but by the time he gave u the letter, the previous week the wife of the secretary to the state government died. So, the governor was mourning and therefore couldn't sign it on time, but it was submitted to the governor's office and started praying that he would sign it. Within that period, the S.S.G.'s wife died, so he was to travel but because of her death, he couldn't, and that made our hope to be brightened again (GOD IS GOOD).

On Saturday morning while in Lagos, we received a massage, which stated that the governor has signed it, and we were very happy and celebrated it.

The next day being Sunday, we went back to my home base in order to get the money.

So, we travelled back on Monday. I was on dialysis and before I could finish, it was very late, so my mum didn't go to their office to collect the money that day. So, on Tuesday, my mum and uncle went for the money and with God on their sides, what should have taken 2-3 days took 1 day (able God). So, on Wednesday, the cheque was collected and everyone were very happy, but the devil was unhappy.

On that same day being Wednesday, in the night around 9pm, after taking my bath and putting on my wears, it was just like an attack, the breathlessness started seriously, and my mum started shouting and praying. She called our landlord and his wife who also joined in the prayers, and immediately, I was rushed to the teaching hospital that night. So, when we got there, I thought I would die to the extent of confessing for the first time. I asked for forgiveness from GOD, my mum, uncle, landlord and my brothers who were there with me. Some people were coming and was consoling my mum thinking I was going to die, even when my uncle went to the village, people were asking him when my mum and relative would bring my corpse for burial, but GOD made me a miraculous child, Praise GOD.

On Wednesday night, I was taken to the theatre, and a surgeon came to put oxygen over my mouth and nose, but to me, it has this unpleasant smell, that I told the surgeon that I didn't need the oxygen. So, the surgeon told the people that came with me, that I wasn't co-operating, and whenever am ready, they should bring me in. When all this were happening, I was almost gone, so they rushed me in and used that same oxygen, but this time the oxygen was used only on my nose.

So, when I was on oxygen, an injection was given to me, and this injection is for me to urinate in order to remove some of the fluid blocking my chest, but unfortunately, I had no kidney, so I didn't urinate. The name of the injection was Lexis.

CHAPTER NINE – The Donor

The doctors gave me so many lexes to the extent that nothing could be done, because they gave me 700mg of it, which was almost the highest. Throughout the night, I was on oxygen, and the doctors said there's nothing they could do. I was so confused, tired and afraid, so I started crying and shouting saying I wanted them to do something, fortunately my elder brother Akachi volunteered to donate kidney to me. So, after some tests by Dr. Ijeoma on compatibility, it was confirmed that it was okay for my brother (Akachi) to donate kidney to me. May God continue to bless him for all his encouragements and for agreeing to donate his kidney.

He came to me and told me that we should do another thing and that thing was prayer. He wanted to hold my hand and I was pushing him away thinking that prayer was a waste of time. He held my hand and we prayed for some time and before the prayer could finish, I felt like vomiting something.

They gave me something like bowel to vomit in it, oh God, I vomited something that is frightening. It looked like intestines to the extent that I thought I vomited my intestines and these were the things blocking my lungs. After the vomiting, I felt so much relief but cough came and each cough precedes blood and mucous and it happened throughout the night in every 5 seconds and these happened around 2am.

I never slept throughout the night rather I was sitting down and by 5am, the thing wanted to start again but I called my elder brother who prayed for me before to come and pray for me again. We prayed for an hour but the continued (God had a plan). The doctors were confused that they told my mum and relatives to prepare and fly me abroad. Before then, my mum called my aunty, my uncle and other relatives to start praying if they wanted me to survive. That night my rev uncle called saying that God told him that nothing will happen to me. After, the doctor told my mum to prepare and take me to Lagos. We waited for an hour before they eventually came and dressed me up. Without brushing my teeth or taking my bath, they took me to the car using a wheel chair.

I, my mum, uncle okey and uncle Ogbonna (he came with us and also came with hand oxygen) who is also a doctor went together. Uncle Ogbonna said it was dangerous to fly me to Lagos because I fly up to 200km above sea level, it would worsen the situation. We decided to go Enugu for dialysis at the teaching Hospital. We called rev Uche I advance to arrange the whole thing while we were still coming and he agreed.

Our movement to Enugu was a tug of war and a very big miracle. In the car, I could not breath (I was gasping for breath). I was uncomfortable with the hand oxygen because it has an unpleasant smell, so I didn't use it for a long time. I thought I was going to die in the car and my mum started crying and praying at the same time.

Uncle Ogbonna also wanted to cry but was praying while uncle okey who was the driver was proclaiming and shouting that I was okay. While they were praying, I started vomiting again into a big water proof which I did till we got to Enugu. Before we got to Enugu, my face turned blue, my veins and arteries all turned blue because there was little or no oxygen in my blood. It was a very terrible experience.

CHAPTER TEN – The Trip to India

When we got to Enugu, I was rushed to the hospital, I was also rushed into the emergency unit where they told me to lie down that oxygen can be placed on me for the meantime because power company took their light and they wanted to buy diesel for the generator set. I couldn't lie don and remember that for about 3-4 hours, I have not lied down, so I had to sit down and take my oxygen. For 4 days, I have not slept and I was sitting down for those days and now, my back was paining me seriously. Sometimes I will fell, my brothers will help and straighten me but I was still in pains. I was there for several hours waiting for the hospital to take the history of what happened to me. In addition, they delayed in buying the diesel for their generator set to the extent that my mum starting begging them to allow her buy the diesel herself but they refused. God still preserved me throughout these hours. As God may have it, in about 4-5 hours of waiting, the light was restored and I was finally taken to the dialysis unit.

Before now, the hospital was on strike and they just resumed so the machine needed to be sterilized very well before use since it has been long, they used it last and also to enhance the efficiency of the machine, so we had to wait for some minutes (about 30 minutes)

After that, I was finally dialyzed but this time for 5 hours. After the dialysis, I felt much better and we went back to my uncle's house to tell him that we had finished. He gave me food but I couldn't eat then because the psychological trauma was much on me, I was just sleeping. Before we could go back to our house, I was almost dark. When we got home, I was told that the S.U fellowship came and prayed for me in my absence against my travelling on Friday and I was also told that my sister came and waited for me but to no avail. When I heard these from my twin brother, I was extremely unhappy. When I came back, I tried to eat a little quantity of food and taking my bath, I was told by my mum that I will be travelling to Lagos the next day. I was extremely sad because I have not told my friends and people dear to me but in all things, I still believed that I had a future and that my future was in Gods hand and that God had a plan for me.

On Friday, I was supposed to take the afternoon flight to Lagos but we came to Enugu late and we couldn't travel that day, we had to sleep at my uncle's house at Enugu. My uncle rev Uche told us not to travel the next day, that we should stay for another dialysis before leaving to avoid what happened earlier, but after looking at the matter, we had to travel that day. But before then, we contacted my aunty at Lagos to prepare for a dialysis center so that I could be dialyzed as soon as I got to Lagos. Our trip was smooth and safe and by 3pm, we were already at Lagos. As soon as we got to Lagos, we started making arrangement for dialysis to avoid what happened earlier.

On that same day, we went to a dialysis center but after looking at the whole thing, we found out that it was costly (36k to 45k). We went to St. Nicholas hospital but on our way, our car spoilt and God helped us in its repair. When we got to the place, we looked at the cost and preferred it. We saw a woman doctor by name Dr. Bamgboye and all arrangements, such as taking down some reports and running of tests. Also, HIV test was conducted that day, and we were asked to come the following day being Sunday by 9am for dialysis. So, the following day, we went back by 9am, as we were instructed. I was dialyzed with a good machine for 4 good hours, and I was better. During the time of dialysis, my mum and uncle Okeh were busy trying to get my visa and ticket. With GOD on their side, they got it on time. I was also dialyzed on Tuesday and Thursday.

My mum spent up to #120,000 for this 3 dialysis at St. Nicholas. So, on Friday, after prayers, we went to Airport which is an international airport by 12 noon and we took off by 2pm (my mom, brother the donor and I)

In the plane, I drank a lot of water, juice, tea and so many things, forgetting that it would affect me. My leg started paining me and also swollen due to the fluid and excess walking which was unavoidable. We travelled from Lagos to Adissababa (Ethiopia capital) to Bombay (Indian capital), and finally to Bangalore (a state in India), but before we could get to India, I was already tired and losing my breath. So, before we could get to Bangalore, we were wondering how we could be able to locate the hospital, since we didn't know our way around India.

As we were coming out from the airport, a man came to ask my brother if he was Uchechukwu from Nigeria, and we said yes, so he helped in carrying our luggage's to the hospital ambulance and we entered with him, and we zoom off to the hospital. When we arrived, I was taken in wheel chair to the doctor's office. They asked my mum some questions, after which I was laid and examined my kidney. They also checked my blood pressure and my weight, and after that I was taken to the ward (Room No 5)

After 30 minutes later, I was taken with a wheel chair to the dialysis unit where they used an access called "jugular catheter" for my dialysis for so many times.

Jugular catheter is a means of getting an access to your blood stream by putting a tube in your neck and leaving it there if you are to transplant but **Vascular access** is getting access to your blood stream using the veins in your hand and it is mainly for people not for transplant, but "Jugular access" is getting access to your blood stream using the veins in your hand. The tube was put in my neck, and was about three weeks there.

That same day, I was dialyzed with a good computerized machine, and it was for 4 hours, and I was told to be drinking less or half of 1 liter a day. Which means that the water I was drink in Nigeria was out of ignorance. The tube was so painful on the first day, but the doctor told me not to worry, that after 2 days, I would be fine. So, after the dialysis, I was taken back to my ward. We were shown the hospital guest house, and my mum met a woman who also came from Nigeria. The woman came with her son named Francis, and after two weeks, the woman cooked, which I found difficult to eat because it was tasteless, but my brother told me it was the best food they could find in Indian. So, I managed to eat small also with the tube pains, also had to manage water too.

They weren't giving me adequate medication, to the extent of going for blood test and x-ray the same day of my arrival and I was also given some drugs. The next two days being Monday, I went for another dialysis, and after which I was taken straight to the ultrasound unit. It was conducted, and the result came out immediately unlike Hansa clinic that took 2-3 days.

I was so strong and had no complications, so that same day I was discharged to go to the guest house, but unfortunately there was no chance there. We were told a woman would be going the next day.

On Wednesday, I went for another one, and we finally headed to the guest house. Francis and I including our donors Anthony and brother Akachi, were going for test in another laboratory, and Francis and his donor were half way to the test because they came before us, and we were just getting started. They were almost through when something tragic happened, along the line one of the tests revealed that the kidney of his donor didn't match with his, and the mother who was to be the attendant became the donor, and they had to start the test afresh, while we were almost through.

I was going for dialysis from the guest house, and the drugs which were given to me made me stronger every day by day, to GOD be the glory.

CHAPTER ELEVEN – The Kidney Transplant

By now people were all confessing that I was stronger on the extent of playing my game and radio on dialysis machine. My dialysis was supposed to be one month before the transplant but mine was 3 weeks and the doctors said that I was fit for the transplant because I had finished my test and all of them were good by Gods grace. By 23rd of march, I was told that my transplant was on the 29th of march being next week Tuesday. That same Wednesday, I was dialyzed and on Saturday I was also dialyzed and they told me to reduce my water intake because any water found in my body will mean that the transplant will no more hold on the proposed date. On Sunday being an Easter Sunday, we went to church for the first time since we came to India. At the church, the devil brought an attack. Every bit of saliva in my tongue finished and my tongue turned white. The plan of the devil was for me to drink water so that the transplant will be affected.

My mum being in confusion told me that we wouldn't go home because we were in the house of the God, so she got some water from the ushers and we went back to the church.

Before the service was over, headache and tiredness came and these two were enough to affect the transplant. When we got to the guest house, my mum was worried, asking God why it was now but by faith I told her that the transplant will still hold on Tuesday. She gave me paracetamol and by morning, I was alright and she was happy.

That Monday 28th, I went for my last dialysis after which, I was on admission waiting for my transplant the next day. By now Francis and his mother who was now the donor were going for series of tests which I have finished undergoing though they came 2 weeks before us. That Monday, in the evening one doctor who happened to be my surgeon, he was the one to fix the draft kidney while another doctor who also came to give me instructions was the person to open it and after fixing, he would close it again.

They told me that I and my brother had to bath ourselves six times with a shampoo they will give us and after which, we should wear our operation dress which they brought. They also told us that starting from 10pm that night, no food or water for us. A woman also came, she is the doctor that would give me the injection for sleeping. She asked me some questions like do you have a girlfriend? Do you smoke or drink?

All these questions made me to shout but she told me that she needed to ask me the questions so that she would not give the wrong injection. When she left, the woman in charge of the wards came and told me not to take my former drugs and she brought "cyclosporine" and game me to prepare the kidney.

By 5 am on the D-day, I and my brother were shaved and we now started waiting for the operation which was supposed to start by 9 am.

By 9am, they came with a stretcher and took my brother and in few minutes, they came and took me and when they were taking me, I looked at my mum and felt like crying. I was taken to a theater where I have never been since I came to India.

When I got in there, I was puzzled by the things I saw there, sophisticated machines for the operation. I was also terrified when I saw the knife, the razor and every other thing that would be used in opening and closing the place. They only thing I did was to start praying and I reminded God of his promise on 25th march. He told me through his word that he would do a new thing. I also told him that I have not been here before and that I commit myself in his hands. After praying, strength and courage came and started waiting for the surgeons. Before the surgeons could be ready, the nurses were preparing the injections and drip to give me.

At last, the surgeons came and one of the surgeons put a tube right inside my bladder to enable me o urinate through the tube after the transplant since I will not be able to move around after the transplant. It was very painful but I endured it because I knew it was my final bus stop by the grace of God. After putting the tube, they brought two planks and fixed it under the surgery bed and placed my hands on them and tied them so I couldn't move my hands and they placed a rectangular rod at a distance and using a cloth to cover it so that I couldn't see what was happening.

That was the only thing I could remember, the next thing I heard was that I should wake up that it was over. Praise the lord.

When I woke up was when I started feeling the pain of the operation and I started shouting and crying, they now took me to the intensive care unit (I.C.U). The I.C.U was a place you will be taken care of and people will not come in there any how and there is a demarcation between the recipient and the people who want to visit them. From there, they will say what they want to say and go. I couldn't do anything on my own. One woman was bathing me and the person that did operation on same day with me. Nobody comes into the I.C.U with his/her shoes or slippers. They gave me a special soap, toothbrush, water, cup, dress and so many things. All these were to prevent infection since my kidney was in a foreign body and is new. A tall and a very beautiful nurse that was taking care of me was fond of me even before the operation. When I came into the I.C.U, I was making her happy by the way I talk with her until we became friends and due to my influence, they started allowing my mum to come and see me in the I.C.U. for 3 days,

I was on drip, I didn't eat anything and, on the 3rd day being a Thursday, I started eating but was still on drip (I took about 12 – 15 drips).

I ate and due to the vacuum created by not eating for 3 days of no food, gas came inside my stomach and for 3 days, I couldn't go to toilet, yet I was still eating food until my stomach started to pain me and every strategy by the nurse to make me to go to toilet failed. On Saturday, the tube that was put in my kidney to filter the blood and the one in my bladder to make me urinate were removed and I was discharged. I was given a mask and taken for ultrasound before I finally went to the ward.

By now, Francis and the donor (mother) were about to finish their tests. The doctor told him that his own transplant will be on Tuesday 8th April 2005. That's a week and 3 days after my own transplant. I stayed about 5 days in the I.C.U being discharged but before i came back to the ward, I was brother was already discharged to go back to the guest house. Every day, they would take blood sample to see if the level of unwanted material in the blood, then were reducing and by the grace of God,

I was. The doctors also come in the morning and they confirmed that I was strong and alright. Even the nurse came around and told me that I was getting better more than the other patients that did transplant same day with me. My weight before I left the I.C.U was 48.6kg and before I left the ward on Monday, the weight was around 49.6kg. when I came the next day for follow up, I was 50.2kg and so on. That is, I started adding weight every day.

On Monday, I was discharged and they told me to be going for a walk (1 hour in the morning and 1 hour in the evening) to enable the wound to heal on time and the fact that my new kidney could be rejected if I dint walk around everyday and often too. I agreed and we went to the guest house after they must have given me my drugs.

CHAPTER TWELVE – The Transplant Patient

When we now got to the guest house, I was eating very well because of the drugs they gave me. I was also going for a walk at a place the doctors said I should go for the purpose. The place is "Around the lake" and by the grace of God, everything was fine. I was undergoing some tests every Tuesday and Thursday and if the doctors see it, they would be very happy because I had no problems before and after the transplant, even Dr. Sundar S who is the managing director and chief nephrologist was very happy. He was happy about my progress in addition to the fact that my weight was increasing (then 57.1kg) and I had a normal renal function and it continued that way. Praise the lord.

By now Francis was very strong and was waiting for Tuesday to come, he was going for dialysis and was growing stronger. By Monday 7th April 2005, he went for final dialysis. The doctor that asked me some series of question before my own transplant also came to him to ask him similar question so as to know the kind of injection to give to him and the preparation was going on but the devil was not happy at all. After the dialysis, he was strong and was taken to the ward for admission as usual, waiting for tomorrow to come. Like an attack he began to have fever, he became sick all of a sudden and the transplant id not hold that day until he got better (Remember, I had my own attack). Instead of getting better, he was getting worse as the days roll by to the extent that his eye was swelling up, his face turned black as if he was dead, his legs were trying to form scales and it was swollen, he was shouting all the time about the pains in his stomach because he couldn't go to toilet, he became thin like a skeleton. This was the person that was stronger than I was before the transplant, and he even went out for shopping himself to the extent of my mum using him for an example, telling me that I should be as strong as he was, now he can't even walk with his legs to the dialysis and he said he was tired. He couldn't even go into the wheel chair himself, the nurses had to carry him and he hardly had the strength to talk, it came to the point that the doctors had to give him some piles of blood just to keep him alive and he was transferred from the room he was to another that had oxygen and he was placed on oxygen.

The mother was so very that she began to slim down and personally I had compassion on her.

One day, my mum went to visit them in the ward, she asked Francis if he was getting better, with his own mouth, he said "NO" and that he was tired. All of these continued for 3 weeks. Before then, we had already booked our flight to return to Nigeria on 2nd may 2005 and the preparation was getting on e.g., undergoing our last test to determine the level of cyclosporine in the blood and other tests to know the number of drugs to give us.

Remember that Dr. Sundar said that he would give us drugs of 3 months and we had to buy for another 3 months which meant that we needed about 2000 dollars to buy the drugs but a miracle happened, after they gave us drugs, it ran up to 7 months but we were looking for 6 months. Praise the lord.

CHAPTER THIRTEEN – The Indian Cow Attack

We were going the hospital everyday for the conclusion e.g., giving us the schedule of drugs, discharge report etc. On Thursday the 28th of April, about 4 days to our departure, around 4pm, we were going to the hospital, we planned in going to a night fellowship from there and my mum was the speaker that day, we had our bibles (the was not happy about our progress and he was trying all he could to stop us). We came to a main road and crossed to the middle of the road and we were waiting for vehicle to pass so that we can cross to the other side of the road, all of a sudden, a cow came and hit me from the back with its horn, as I was falling, I dragged my mum and fell down on the road and thank God no vehicle was coming because Indian driver are very rough in driving. I know that the plan of the devil was to get me so wouldn't be able to go on Monday the next week or my draft kidney to be damaged when we fell down. The people there didn't move to help us at all and they saw what happened instead, some of them was laughing at us. Immediately, we stood up but my mother's hand was swollen, we went back straight to the doctors and after seeing it, they referred us to the doctor in the orthopedics. After the x-ray, it was discovered that a small bone broke in my mums' hand i.e., she had a fracture. A plaster was out on her which she was to carry for a week, she was very unhappy and I was crying silently. The doctor prescribed some drugs for us and we bought it and every pain was going down gradually and because the drugs, the pain that my mum was having due to the fact that she fell in the bathroom years ago was relieving too, maybe it was one of the plans of God for allowing the thing to happen. That day, we couldn't go to the fellowship again but we called the pastor and told him what happened.

Everyone that saw it, thanked God for not allowing it to happen to me because it would have been tragic and not allowing a vehicle to be coming on that side that I fell into, and my mum thanked God because absolutely, nothing happened to me, not even a scratch. Praise the lord. I just thank God for relieving the pain on time because when it newly happened, it really pained her so much that she couldn't sleep at night and I was crying because she was uncomfortable. Praise be to God for everything.

CHAPTER FOURTEEN – The Return to Nigerian

After 3 weeks of Francis tragedy, on the 4th week, he was getting stronger and that was the week the accident happened. The doctors now told him that his own transplant will be on 29th April 2005 being on Friday, exactly one month that I did mine and everyone was happy, and we praised God, sang and prayed to the glory of God. Amen. On 29th the D-day, we went in with a family that came for check up and prayed, sang and encouraged Francis, telling him that it would soon be over and we left.

That day, God helped us a lot, we settled almost everything e.g., our drugs, our reports, and the doctor bidding us goodbye and good luck. My mum also went to a dentist because one of her teeth was shaking and he gave her drugs and we also went to the diabetologist because she had diabetics and she was given drugs and her own was also settled and we started waiting for Monday but we went back to the guest house. We went to see how Francis and the mother was doing, both of them were in the I.C.U but the mum was still unconscious, and Francis was in serious pains, shouting and crying and both of them were on oxygen but we just thanked God that the transplant was successful and we knew that the pain would be over soonest.

We now went home, packed my drugs and other things and we were now waiting for Monday. Praise the Lord. I want you know that if you trust God, believe in his word and he will never abandon you. The bible says "I will have mercy upon whom I will have mercy"

Believe with me that God says yes, nobody can say no not even the devil. I urge you to stand firm even in the time of difficulties because he is the author and finisher of our faith. If you've not surrendered or given your life to Christ, tomorrow may be too late, please accept Jesus and you will never regret it, he will always be there for you. Trials and temptations might/must come but my God is a perfect God and he will provide a way of escape for you. "Trust GOD and see the sweetness in knowing him but remember, he has a purpose for everything"

My dear readers, God is really good, we went all the way from India on air with no problems and when we came to Lagos, my Aunties and Uncles saw me and were extremely happy that I came back health and strong. My aunty by name Ngozi found It difficult to remove her eyes on me because she saw how fat I was and how I started doing the things I never did for some months. They praised and thanked God for his preservation there at India, protection as in his journey mercies upon us from Nigeria to India and back to Nigeria.

We had to spend about one and half days in air, we left India by 4pm on Monday 2nd May 2005 and we came back to Nigeria on 3rd May 2005 but I thank God personally who never allowed to encounter any problems on the way, may his name be blessed. Amen.

On Wednesday, we came back home my friends were already waiting for my arrival – Ogbuzuru, Oluchi, Friday, Nkiruka to mention but a few and I wasn't happy that my sister wasn't there but I know she had a reason for that. I was happy when they shouted for joy and praised God for his healing and then, I knew I was loved by many. I pray that God will bless all of them in Jes us name. Amen. After my arrival, many people visited me and they also praised God for what he has done for me.

I believe that all that happened, came to happen so that God will make a name for himself and I thank God that his name was finally praised though it wasn't the will of the devil. I also thank God for what he told my uncle on that Wednesday that I almost passed on. He said that "the sickness wasn't unto death but to the glory of God" says the lord and the lord honored his word by healing me. I also bless his name because when the whole thing started on 1st January 2005, when blood filled my mouth at abut 6am, my mum started the with tears and crying but I said to myself "since my mum started the year with tears, she would end the year with extreme joy" and God have honored my word by healing me. Blessed be the name of God because during the time of my illness, my mum was very thin and was looking like an old woman but I thank God because my mum has regained all that she lost during my illness. She now became fat to the extent that her dresses which very loosen on her when I was sick, now became very tight and uncomfortable on her when I became alright and I praise God for that.

I also want to thank God because when I was sick, my mum was contemplating whether I will take my JAMB, WAEC, NECO exams, but I bless God that all of them was registered for me due to the faith in my mum and everybody in my family. I bless God that I came back and still et all of them, I mean the three of them. I know that I never read since December last year (2004) until the time I came into the exam hall, but many of my classmates were coming to me for me to teach them mathematics (remember that I was not there when it was taught). I taught them and they were saying that I was reading when I was still in India but the truth was that I never read there in India, in fact I was not with any of my textbooks and I had no time to read after all, I was uncomfortable because of the things that was in my blood before my transplant, so how could I have read? But I know that it's not because I am very intelligent but its just the grace of the most high God.

I bless the name of the most high God for making me to be faithful even in the exam hall, he never allowed me to engage in any form of examination malpractice, I know everything in the paper, but I believe that all these were the grace of God. May His Name be blessed. Amen.

My dear readers, if you still don't believe that our God is a miracle God, then you must be a very big mistake somewhere, so the earlier you start believing, the better for you. I am saying this out of experience. Always know that everything that happens in your life works for good but, provided you love God by obeying him.

I am calling my God, the God of miracle because when I was in pains, a visitor came, and my grandmother was telling the visitor that anytime I am being prayed for, the sickness would get worse, making the prayer warriors to get down in faith. I was in the sitting room when she said that, and I told her not to worry that I would definitely bounce back, and you would be the first to dance, though I was in a serious pain when I was saying that to her.

I sure know that when a snake is killed, before it dies it intend to roll itself with all its last strength before dying. That is what happened in my case. The devil came with all his last strength, because he knows he has been defeated. All these powers he is showcasing was a manipulation to make the prayer warrior decline in faith, so as to continue his operation in my life, but God never allowed that to come to pass, instead he was motivating them to pray harder, may His Name be praised Amen.

My dear readers, let me tell you that when something is happening to you, and you pray instead of the problem vanishing, it increases, but don't decline in prayers. Pray harder because God has heard you, but the devil will make you believe that God doesn't answer prayers. Again, stand firm in the Lord, and remember that when our Master Jesus Christ was casting out demons, the bible says that the demons tormented the person possessed by them, and the person would fall down and begin to roll. Some people must have thought that Jesus was a fake healer, that instead of his prayer making things better, it is making it worse, but the truth is that he has won the devil, and he has begun to showcase all his last powers, for he knows that his inhabitant has been taken away from him by a more superior Master, and he was doing it to make the faith of the prayer warriors to decline, but God never allowed it to happen like that, rather he instituted into them more power and strength to fight the last battle.

I bless the Lord because when I came back from Lagos to my home base on the 3rd of May 2005, I was still in the car when I saw my grandmother dancing, and she was d only person that danced on my return, meaning that God honored my word.

I also want to thank God for my life, because I have heard so many stories of people that died on dialysis machine, but my great redeemer saved my soul from all the dialysis I did, even when they were complications on some occasions that was enough to make me pass on, but God saved me, may His name be blessed. I also thank God for the kind of friends he gave me, who mourned with me when I was sick, and rejoiced with me when I was healed. I bless God for people like Oluchi, Ifeoma, Friday, Chinasa, Nonso, Obinna, Nkechi, Nkiru, Alice and so many of them who visited and prayed for me during the time of my sickness, to the extent of leaving school during school hours and visiting me to make sure that I was alright. I won't forget people like Ogonna, Nneamaka, Chika, Ugochi, Amarachi her sister, Nnenna, Ifeanyi, Chukwuemeka, Okechukwu and Victor. In fact, I don't even know how to mention all that were there for me during the time of my sickness.

I want to tell you that as far as you re a child of God, when you speak a word, it shall be so, as far as you believe it. I am saying it because I made some declarations when I was sick, I was being prayed for, and after prayers, the sickness became worse, my mum came and asked me why I was making her faith to go down and I reminded her of what happened at the Hospital, and how I was kept in a room where people that are supposed to die, and how I suffered there. I said to her, mum when all these shall be over, you will be the first to laugh. I am telling you that immediately I came out of the theatre. I was still in the stretcher, and they were taking me to I.C.U. I saw my mum and waved my hands at her, and she smiled and laughed at the same time, therefore my word was honored by God Almighty.

Another was that when we went to India and we knew that we were supposed to go back to India for check-up after six months of my discharge from the hospital and in effect, we were supposed to have six months drugs or medication to sustain me till those six months, we now found out that we paid for 3 months drugs and not six months and I believe that God made us to notice so late so as make nae for himself.

We were discussing with people that came for check-up and in the cause of our discussion, we now found out that mistake, my mum became very confused that she never knew what to do because the remaining drugs can cost up to 2000 dollars which my mum didn't have and have no hope of getting anywhere. She called my uncle several times to tell him of our predicament and asked him (uncle Uche) to send at least 1500 dollars to us so as to complete the drugs but unfortunately, my uncle told her that he has no such money but he will try and find it because it is not easy to return to India after 3 months of our discharge i.e., it is very costly.

To add salt to our already existing injury, those that came for check-up also told us that since we spent one month after my transplant, that Dr Sundar will give us only 2 months medication and this made my mum to be confused even more. In that situation, I am the one to be worried but on the contrary, I was not disturbed because I knew that the Almighty God can never abandon any project half way.

I believed within me that since God saved me from the kidney failure and a kidney transplant which was more deadly and dangerous, that my drugs are just a simple matter to him, after all, silver and gold are his, so I was not afraid. In the cause of my mum's confusion, I told her not to worry and made a proclamation "Mum do you see this drug you are worried about? We are going to go with more than the required medication". Humanly speaking, my told thought that I spoke like a child after considering the condition surrounding us but I knew what my God could do.

The next time that my mum called my uncle, he now promised to send 1000 dollars to us and that was the first miracle but my mum wasn't satisfied with it but I also told her not to worry. Secondly, we came to the hospital for check-up and the director by name Dr Sundar told us that he would give us 6 months medication instead of 3 months. My mum wanted to be happy but I told her to stand still and see the salvation of the lord.

Thirdly, we went to the hospital for check-up and same doctor promised to add one-month drugs to our medication but I told my mum that I wasn't yet complete, and at last the 1000 dollars from my uncle arrived and they now gave us my drugs. After cross checking everything, we found out that it was 7 months drugs and not 6 months again. God honored my word, Praise the Lord.

I want to thank God because I know it was not the will of the devil for me to come back that Monday that we intended to come back for a reason. As said earlier, On 28th may being Thursday, we were concluding our last days in India, we were going to the hospital in the evening for the arrangement of our drugs and from there we were supposed to go to fellowship where my mum was supposed to be the speaker, we came to the middle of the main road, we stood waiting for the vehicles on the other side of the road to pass and suddenly a Cow from nowhere came and hit us with the horn at my back and the velocity of the hit made me to fly and I jumped on my mum and we both fell on the main road, to God be the glory that no car was coming, if not, nobody knows what could have happened to us but God saved us out of the abundance of his love.

According to my mum, the cow had ring on its horn signifying that I wasn't an ordinary cow. We were saying maybe the demonized cow must have seen our bible and also our progress in other people's land but Jesus has always been the winner. Praise the lord. I want to thank because had it been I had any injury, it could have affected my kidney and it could have been a very big battle but God never allowed it to happen.

Though mum had fracture on her hand (the bone of her wrist), we went to the orthopedic and something like plaster was fixed and that night my mum cried and she never knew how to sleep as the fracture was paining her so much and I never knew what to do that night but to cry with her.

I bless God that all that is now a story we are telling for the glory of the lord and I bless God that nothing happened to both of us even my elder brother Akachi who came back to Nigeria roughly 2 weeks after my transplant, God almighty protected him even when the injury caused by the transplant wasn't healed but God saw him through and gave him a safe journey back to Nigeria, may his name be blessed, Amen.

I also want to bless the name of the almighty God and my purposeful Jehovah for what he did on the 26th of April 2005, when we wanted to go for fellowship and we went to the pastors house by name pastor Gavin from where we will go with another elder in the church to the fellowship venue, from Asaye road where the quest house was situated to the cuck bund road where the pastors house was located, we boarded an auto rick Shaw popularly known as "Keke napep" with our bibles and other materials like my drugs and handset, we came down thinking that we came down with everything but after some minutes of coming down from the rickshaw, I found out that I forgot my bible in that place. I was extremely unhappy, uncomfortable and restless. I started looking for it even in the flower inside the pastors' compound, my mum told me not to worry and that I wasn't my fault after all nobody is above mistake or forgetting something anytime and anyplace but I was not satisfied with her words instead I went to the main road looking for the rickshaw man to drove us to the place, but sadly I never saw him again, so I had no choice than forgetting about it and leaving everything in the hands of the lord.

I went into the pastor house and he told me that he understands how I feel, but that I shouldn't worry that my bible has gone for a greater evangelism somewhere.

I knew that God wanted to do something because everything works for a purpose as far as God is concerned. A day before the Tuesday of the sad occurrence, I put one of my passports in my bible but truly speaking, I can't tell what pushed me to do that, I guess it the Lord doing and on Wednesday 27th April 2005, that rickshaw man brought my bible back to the guest house. I was extremely happy and my mum was glad, we thanked the man so much and appreciated him with 100 rupees and the bible came back to me. Praise the lord.

So, my reader and friend, trust in the lord with your whole understanding of what he can do and in all your ways acknowledge him and he shall direct your path. What is it that you think is your problem that the lord can't give you?

Is it a problem of sickness? I believe it is not as bad as mine. Don't you think that God can heal you? Be it physical, emotional, spiritual and psychological?

Of course, he can. I Uchechukwu miracle Kalu-Orji is telling you that he will visit you at that point. Is it money? The bible says that "silver and gold are mine" says the lord, he will surely visit you as far as you are his child just trust him and believe in him.

My dear, is it spiritual problem? You will want to stand but you will see yourself going back, firmness is of the lord coupled with your willingness to serve him. I am telling you not to get weak, don't draw back, continue I prayer, if it is your will to serve God but your flesh is your limitation, ask God to lift you up and make you stand on the solid rock which is Jesus Christ, and I tell you of a truth and out of experience that God whose mercies and love is forevermore will answer you. Remember that he said that it is no his will that any body should perish but come to repentance. Salvation is a choice and since you have chosen to serve God, he will never abandon you for he created you in his image and likeness.

Is it that you think that you can't give your life to Christ because you think there is no gain there? I pity for you because you refused to acknowledge your father and your savior who died to set you free from eternal death in hell fire.

Remember that heaven is real and hell fire is also real but the choice is yours, and know you that your decision affects your future and where you will spend your eternity after life. There are billions of people in hell gnashing their teeth and wishing they had the opportunity you have to hear the word of God even if it was once but here you are playing with your life. "Jesus is coming soon". My dear, that thing you think you are enjoying will soon roll away and you are preparing a special room for yourself in hell fire "WHAT SHALL IT PROFIT A MAN TO GAIN THE WHOLE WORLD AND LOSE HIS OWN SOUL" meditate on the word of God and repent today, remember "tomorrow may be too late" Jesus loves you so much.

Are you a child of God? Hold fast to that which you have for there is a great reward for you in heaven, not only that every of your needs shall be provided "God will provide all your needs according to his riches in glory". Your father is the king of kings and the lord of lords.

Know you that silver and gold belong to the lord and heaven, earth and everything in it is his. So why are you worried about what you need and you have not gotten it, have faith in him and he will establish it to the glory of his name. if the sons and daughters of governors and presidents do no lack anything as far as money and other physical things are concerned, yet their peace is limited, how much the governor of all governors and the president of all presidents who happen to be your father in heaven.

Do you think you will lack anything? Of course not, you will not lack anything just fear the lord, trust in him, have faith and believe that he will do it for you, and most importantly, be patient.

"O fear the lord you saints, for there is no lack for them that fear him" Psalms 34:9. Just pray and tell God that your problem with faith and in the name of Jesus Christ and it is already yours. O ye child of God, try I today and prove the lord a just God. Do it today.

Are you passing through temptation as a child of God? Do not worry, it is the will of God for you to be strong in him. Remember that our lord Jesus Christ said that since we believe in him that the world will definitely hate us and persecute us and also remember that "No temptation has taken you except that which is common to man" and God is faithful for he will not allow us to be tempted more than we can bear but, in the temptation, he will provide a way of escape, that way we may be able to bear it. (1 Corinthians 10:13), also read Psalm 34:19. O you child of God, don't doubt God, don't even doubt his faithfulness. Know you that he will always be there to hear your prayers Psalm 34:15. The only thing you need is to take heed to these nine keys to success in the lord (Spiritual Victory)

1. Key of forgiveness from God and men
2. Patience
3. Fellowship in Jesus always
4. Faithfulness and purity
5. Fasting and prayer
6. Key od spotlessness
7. Faith and praise
8. Entire consecration
9. Holiness which is the master key.

As you do it, God bless you. Amen.

CHAPTER FIFTEEN – The Thanksgiving and Testimonies

This happens to be one of my proclamations while I was sick and in pains. Now, I happens to be the most memorable of all the proclamations I ever made in that period of suffering. One day when my breathlessness and restlessness was extremely serious, and I was to be rushed to Agani road Enugu for dialysis, my brother chia carried me on his back to the car for I couldn't walk, when we got to the car, in pains, restlessness, discomfort and breathlessness, I said tom my mum "mummy, do know that, that day will be great" she was confused and asked me which day and I simply said "the day of my thanksgiving". She never knew what to say maybe because she thought I was speaking like a child but I knew that I saw that be the inspiration of the holy spirit, so that God's name shall be glorified, even on that day, my mum never knew whether to say amen or to say ok or to just keep quiet. The quietness was caused by her emotional and physical state due to my illness but I meant what I was saying but she didn't understand.

I want to bless God for honoring my word on the 19th of June 2005.Remember that in this June,

I added a name to my already existing name "MIRACLE". Because of all the things God has done for me and all the miracles he did for me, he gave a name "Miracle" which I believe shall follow me all the days of my life in Jesus name. when we came back, we were planning on how to run some tests for my health according to the instructions the Indian doctors gave us. They told us to be going for some test weekly and monthly depending on the things to be found in the tests and all the results should be forwarded to them via E-mail. One day the doctor that saw me by name Dr. Kidi, asked my uncle – Ogbonna who happens to be a doctor in same hospital if I was still alive and my uncle said "Yes", that I was transplanted and that I am back to town and he shouted and said he wanted to see me with his eyes, he was very surprised because he saw and understood my condition then. That night he came to the house, saw me and gave thanks to God and also appreciated my brother who donated his kidney (bro Akachi).

On one of the occasions when we went to hospital for test, another doctor who saw me that night never recognized me because I changed for the better. When he was hearing the kind of test I came to do, and the mask I was putting on to prevent diseases and infections, he had t ask question if I was the person and we said yes. He never knew what to say but he told my "your son is destined to live".

These were all the testimonies, when all these started newly, as in when I went to the hospital at Enugu, where they didn't take good care of me; later after my recovery, my grand mum accompanied by my uncle Uche, went to the hospital for my grand mum check-up and one of the nurses that saw me while I was on admission asked my uncle whether I was still alive and my uncle said yes and she shouted because they thought I was going to die but they never knew my God. As God may have, great were the testimonies that was told because of God's miracles in my life and to the glory of his name. May his name be blessed and adored above other names. Amen.

About the Thanksgiving Day, I was a very happy and memorable day for every member of my family and it was done in accordance to my proclamation. The preparation of the thanksgiving was very fantastic. They program and the invitation card were all computerized and beautiful. Even the executive governor of our state was supposed to be the special guest of honor and his wife the mother of the day. It even attracted the attention of the general superintendent of our church Rev Charles, who was supposed to be the speaker of the day but as God may have it, he brought the people of his choice. The governor and wife were represented by the wife to the deputy governor Mrs. Catherine and rev Charles represented by the men's' president general council. My thanksgiving attracted so many personalities, so many commissioners, both new and old ones came, permanent secretaries, so many ministers of God, both from far and near including our pastor at the village, many local government chairmen and secretaries came and many people came on the 19th June 2205. Many E.C members of our church came to the extent that the moderator was Rev Okeh and prayer directed by the district superintendent of our church also honored the invitation, in fact, I was great. My classmates and my friends in the fellowship and school came to the thanksgiving service to the extent that I was very happy and extremely overwhelmed with joy and gladness. Some of them were Nnenna, my sister Ifeoma, her sister Ugochi and Amarachi, Uche, Chukwudi, Chinasa, Oluchi, Awada, Nkiru, Alice and most of the Excos pf the scripture Union 2004/2005 session and 2005/2006 session with

Ogonna and Ugochi being the president of the two sessions. In fact, I don't know what to say but God bless them. Even the people I didn't event invite and I never knew their names. So many people came even girls from my mum's school came. In fact, I don't really know how to explain the greatness of the day but the day was really great.

The preaching by Rev. Azuka made people to give their life to Christ and God was glorified, meaning that the was really great both physical and spiritual because was happy over the souls that were saved. The church was decorated, we danced the dance of joy, I got a surprise package by the way my friends honored my invitation and how we danced to the glory of God.

Food was fantastic, 4 to 5 goats including a ram were bought just for the occasion. So many things were cooked (fried rice, garri, jollof rice, chicken, pepper soup and so many things that I can't remember). The people that sang did it wonderfully and the people were invited from Umuahia by my brother Akachi and they sang till we were tired of dancing. That day was great, praise the lord.

So, my dear, a I want to conclude this writing, I would want to ask you, do you still believe in God? Or are you still doubting him? If you have not given your life to God, I pity you and I am praying for you and will continue praying for you. A king in heaven that created men came down, and died in the hands of them that he created just to save you from eternal death oh, what a love? And why do you want to crucify him the second time. My dear, if you still a sinner, repent and give your life to the almighty Jesus who died for you. Do it today for tomorrow may be too late.

If you are a child of God, always believe miracle is your right because Jesus said that "signs and wonders shall follow them that believe" and since you are believer healing, prosperity, miracle, protection, provision, guidance, presence of the lord shall be with you as far as you continue being faithful to God. Whatsoever you may be passing through, God is aware of that and he has a purpose for everything. God bless you all. Amen.

CHAPTER SIXTEEN – THE GLORIOUS END

If you have come this far, that simply means you want to know the end of the story. All the chapters before this chapter were all written by my brother himself, Uchechukwu. However, this particular chapter was written by me, Obinna.

This chapter will tell you the ending of the story. My brother started the story, but then life happened.

It's a sad story, but we give God all the glory. If not for God, I wonder how it would have ended. Though it ended this way however, we are still grateful to God for bringing us this far, for helping us through all the challenges.

After the dedication, the dedication actually happened in 2005. That was when the kidney transplant took place.

My brother traveled to India for the transplant. The transplant was actually successful. My brother by name, Akachukwu, donated his kidney.

The transplant was successful. The traveling was successful. The money for the transplant by God's grace was made available.

After the transplant, they came back and our lives continued normally. however, my brother had to be taking drugs continuously for everything to come to normalcy. He has to be taking that because normally after transplant, you're supposed to be taking drugs for the wound to heal.

Everything was normal again. After a few months, the situation of the kidney failure came back again. This is a situation that everybody couldn't explain.

Is it that the transplant was not done very well, or the drugs made it to fail again, or the kidney wasn't matching, or what? nobody could explain what happened. The only thing we could remember was that the new kidney failed again. It was actually disheartening, very, very disheartening however, who are we to question God? My brother titled his book, God's Will. If you check it closely, you still notice that it is truly God's Will.

God gave my brother the opportunity to reunite with his people, you see, to probably make his way straight.

Don't worry. Listen up. You understand why I said to make his ways straight.

Now, when the situation came back again, we as humans, tried to manage the situation. Mind you, we've already spent a lot of money to come this far.

At the peak of the sickness, we were doing dialysis. For you to manage a kidney failure, you'll be doing dialysis. Dialysis is a situation where you have to filter the urine in the blood, because the kidneys' work is to filter the urine in the blood.

Normally, urine mixes with the blood, but then the kidneys' work is to remove that urine from the blood. That urine that is in the blood, if left in the blood, is enough to cause a lot of damage to the body. So, the kidneys' work is to filter the urine from the blood.

You see, anytime I see people smoking, they don't know the kind of damage it is doing to their liver.

Normally, there are some habits that are so habitual that, even if you want to stop it, it becomes difficult for you to stop it.

I know that you are still in charge. You can stop some habits. I had a particular habit that I was able to stop.

If somebody told me that I'll be able to stop that habit, I'll tell you it's a lie. It seemed impossible to stop however, I was able to stop it.

So, I'm encouraging you today. That habit of smoking, that habit of too much alcohol, that habit of beating a woman, that habit of fighting unnecessarily, that habit of claiming rights, when you should have settled issues with dialogue, you can stop it. It's your choice.

You have the power to stop it. You see, that part of your body is valuable. Smoking destroys the liver over time.

You can stop it. If that liver fails, bringing it back will be very difficult. This is your chance to turn back.

Back to the story. When the problem came back again, we tried to manage the situation. We were doing dialysis.

This dialysis, at that time wasn't a small amount of money. This dialysis we are talking about is not done once a week. Sometimes, you need to do it three or minimum two times a week. This was money involving.

Another thing, where we do the dialysis is some kilometers away from where we live. It wasn't a close distance. Sometimes, it will just come at once and we will all enter the car and rush.

Probably, when we are on our way, it will probably be when we will be searching for the fund. Thank God for everything. We managed it for some time, but then it came to a point that we couldn't manage it again.

On our way to the dialysis center on a faithful day, we were inside our car. We were actually close to the dialysis center. That's when my brother noticed that he couldn't make it again.

He tried. He fought.He tried all he could, but then he couldn't make it again. Before he gave up, he dropped a sentence for me that keeps ringing in my heart till now. He spoke with assurance and he told me something.

He said, Obinna, **we will meet in heaven**. Do you know what that means? That's a strong sentence. Obinna, **see you in heaven**.

With that kind of assurance, we will see in heaven. The assurance was so strong. Anytime I live my life careless, I will just be like, Obinna, you need to change your ways.

That word is like a continuous evangelism to me. It keeps ringing in my heart.

Obinna, you have a place you should be. Mend your ways. Turn back.to God Always do the right thing so that you'll be in this heaven. Do you know what it means? **"Obinna, we'll see in heaven."**

So, this is still like an evangelism to you. We will see in heaven. It's possible.

It's possible. You and I can be in heaven. We can make it.

All we need is to turn away from sin. It's not always easy, but if you yield yourself to God, you can make it. Christ died for us.

He gave us hope of tomorrow. He gave us hope of resurrection. That's to tell you that life does not end after death.

Some people think that once you die, that's the end. That's not the end. Once you are born, you are born.

You continue to live. The only thing you drop is your body. You drop your skin, but then there is still soul.

There is still spirit. You have three in you. You have the body; you have the soul and you have the spirit.

The spirit is the spirit of God. The body is the sand. God made us with the sand.

Mend your ways. Live daily prepared for that eternity. There is heaven and there is hell. Choose your destination right by living a good life.

Don't think that everything starts and ends on earth. That's why some people can have the boldness to take their lives. What you don't give, you don't take. You cannot give yourself your life. So by default, you're not supposed to take your own life because you are not the person that gave yourself life. So you shouldn't take your own life. If you take your own life, you're already giving yourself a ticket to hell.

Let me tell you, my brother and my sister, there is heaven and there is hell. Where you go to is determined by what you do now that you are still alive. Now that you are alive, you have the ability to decide on some things however, once you are dead, you don't have the ability to make any decision.

This is your opportunity to make the decision of having access to heaven. This is the opportunity you have to make that particular decision, the decision of turning back to God, the decision of keeping your ways straight at all and the decision of remaining rapturable at all time.

May the help us to remain rapturable at all time in Jesus' name, Amen.

APPRECIATION

The bible says that in everything, give thanks to him. Even in times of trouble, he is there to save us. He does things in a perfect time and in a perfect way. Likewise, I am saying to this most excellency, may all glory, all honor, all adoration be ascribed to him now and forevermore, Amen. I just want to thank God for the people who he used in different dimension to see me through. May God bless and provide all their needs according to his riches in glory through Christ Jesus our lord, Amen.

First of all, I want to thank my mum who has always been there for me, what a loving and caring mother indeed, with all the sleepless night, she was always there to comfort me when in pains. I know that I cannot do enough to thank her but by the grace of God, I will try my best to make her happy. May God see her through in all aspects of life, she never ceased praying for me.

I want to thank my elder brother – Akachi, who voluntarily donated his kidney to me. A decision like that is not always an easy one to take.

If not for him agreeing to donate his kidney to me, I probably wouldn't be alive to write this story up to this point. I pray that may the Lord guide and keep him always in Jesus name. Amen.

I also want to thank my twin brother – Obinna, who helped me a lot by comforting me, telling me that everything will be alright, not minding the fact that sometimes I make him not to go to school, but thanks to God that he was always there when I needed him the most. May God bless him for me.

Furthermore, I thank God for my Uncle Okeh, who left his family at Lagos to be with us. He helped in pursuing almost all the formalities concerning our travelling to India like getting our international passport, getting our visa, yellow fever, even our tickets. He also helped in transporting us to almost everywhere we went to due to the fact that my mum cannot drive then due to the confusion, God bless you

I will not forget my uncle – Uche for the calls and connections he made towards my kidney transplant. I really appreciate them all and o pray that God will continue to guide and protect him and his family now and always in Jesus' name, Amen.

www.ingramcontent.com/pod-product-compliance
Lightning Source LLC
Chambersburg PA
CBHW071420210526
45465CB00001B/474